Healthy Keto Air Fryer Cooking Plan

A Complete Keto Air Fryer Cookbook to Stay Fit & Healthy

Lucy Grant

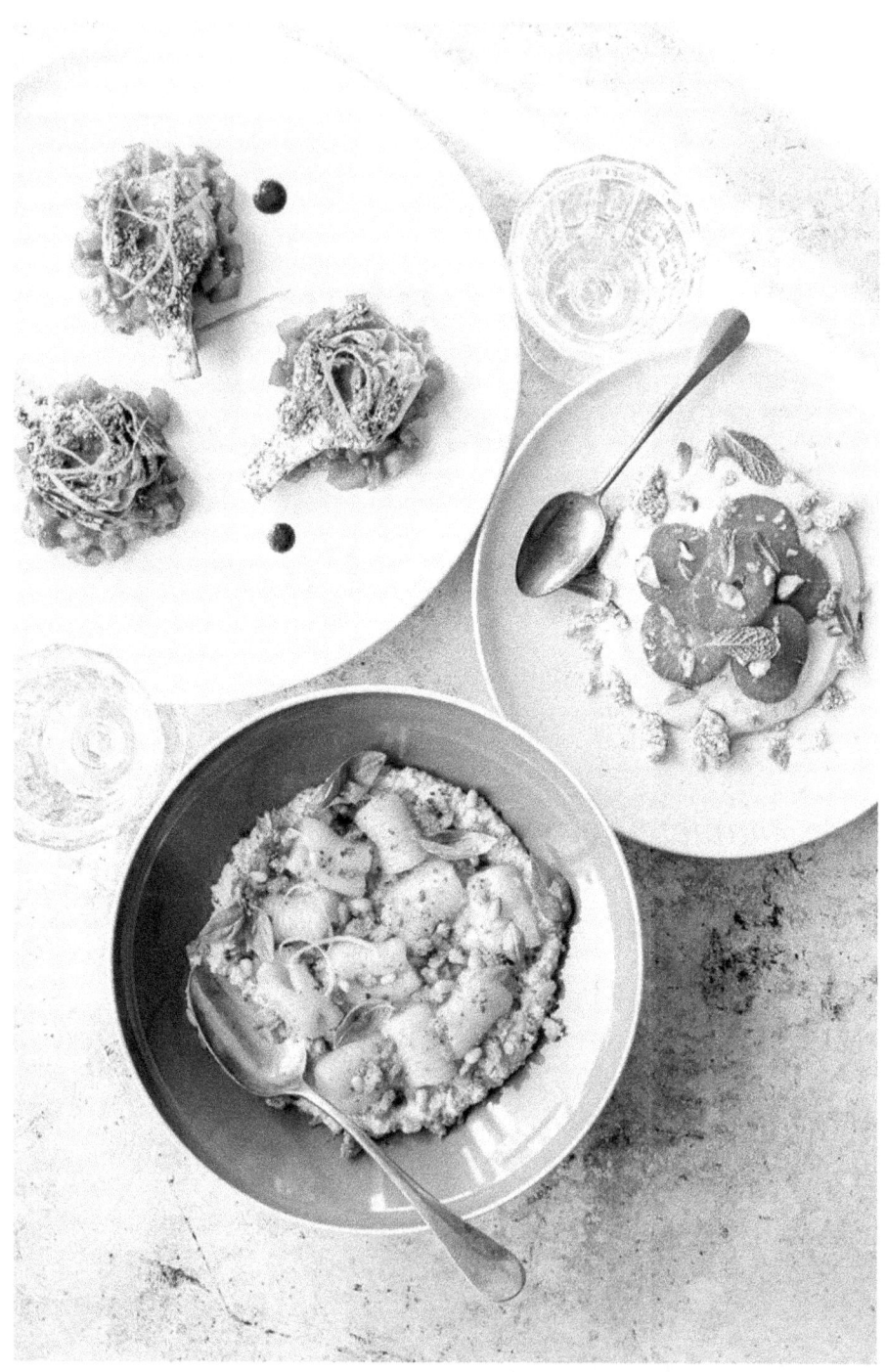

© Copyright 2020 All rights reserved.

The following Book is reproduced below with the goal of providing information that is as accurate and reliable as possible. Regardless, purchasing this Book can be seen as consent to the fact that both the publisher and the author of this book are in no way experts on the topics discussed within and that any recommendations or suggestions that are made herein are for entertainment purposes only. Professionals should be consulted as needed prior to undertaking any of the action endorsed herein.

This declaration is deemed fair and valid by both the American Bar Association and the Committee of Publishers Association and is legally binding throughout the United States.

Furthermore, the transmission, duplication, or reproduction of any of the following work including specific information will be considered an illegal act irrespective of

if it is done electronically or in print. This extends to creating a secondary or tertiary copy of the work or a recorded copy and is only allowed with the express written consent from the Publisher. All additional right reserved.

The information in the following pages is broadly considered a truthful and accurate account of facts and as such, any inattention, use, or misuse of the information in question by the reader will render any resulting actions solely under their purview. There are no scenarios in which the publisher or the original author of this work can be in any fashion deemed liable for any hardship or damages that may befall them after undertaking information described herein.

Additionally, the information in the following pages is intended only for informational purposes and should thus be thought of as universal. As befitting its nature, it is presented without assurance regarding its prolonged validity or interim quality. Trademarks that are mentioned are done without written consent and can in no way be considered an endorsement from the trademark holder.

Table of Contents

CRISPY CROUTONS 10

ROASTED ASPARAGUS WITH SERRANO HAM 12

VERY BERRY BREAKFAST PUFFS 14

CHICKEN SUN-DRIED TOMATOES & MUSHROOMS 16

BBQ MEATLOAF 18

DELICIOUS CHICKEN FAJITA CASSEROLE 20

CREAMY SPINACH 22

BROCCOLI NUGGETS 25

CAULIFLOWER TOMATO RICE 27

CHEESY ZUCCHINI NOODLES 30

CHEESE BAKED BROCCOLI 34

STUFFED BELL PEPPERS 36

DELICIOUS ZUCCHINI CASSEROLE 38

PARMESAN SQUASH CASSEROLE 41

PECAN GREEN BEAN CASSEROLE 43

BRUSSELS SPROUTS AND BROCCOLI 45

BASIL EGGPLANT CASSEROLE 47

SPICY OKRA 49

AIR FRY ASPARAGUS 51

CRISP BRUSSELS SPROUTS 53

TASTY CAULIFLOWER RICE 55

SPINACH SQUARES 58

VEGETABLE KEBABS 60

BLACKENED TILAPIA 62

GARLIC BUTTER BAKED SHRIMP 65

CAJUN CATFISH FILLETS 67

LEMON GARLIC SHRIMP 70

COD WITH VEGETABLES 73

HEALTHY SWORDFISH FILLETS 75

AIR FRY FISH PATTIES 77

DELICIOUS SHRIMP FAJITAS 79

TASTY CRAB PATTIES 82

CAJUN SCALLOPS 84

GREEK BAKED SALMON 86

WHITE FISH FILLET WITH ROASTED PEPPER 89

ROSEMARY BASIL SALMON 91

TOMATO BASIL FISH FILLETS 93

BAKED SALMON & CARROTS 95

BAKED SHRIMP SCAMPI 97

TANGY SALMON 99

CHEESE HERB SALMON 101

CRISPY COCONUT SHRIMP 104

Introduction

What's the difference between an air fryer and deep fryer? Air fryers bake food at a high temperature with a high-powered fan, while deep fryers cook food in a vat of oil that has been heated up to a specific temperature. Both cook food quickly, but an air fryer requires practically zero preheat time while a deep fryer can take upwards of 10 minutes. Air fryers also require little to no oil and deep fryers require a lot that absorb into the food. Food comes out crispy and juicy in both appliances, but don't taste the same, usually because deep fried foods are coated in batter that cook differently in an air fryer vs a deep fryer. Battered foods needs to be sprayed with oil before cooking in an air fryer to help them color and get crispy, while the hot oil soaks into the batter in a deep fryer. Flour-based batters and wet batters don't cook well in an air fryer, but they come out very well in a deep fryer.

The ketogenic diet is one such example. The diet calls for a very small number of carbs to be eaten. This means food such as rice, pasta, and other starchy vegetables like potatoes are off the menu. Even relaxed versions of the keto diet minimize carbs to a large extent and this compromises the goals of many dieters. They end up having to exert large amounts of willpower to follow the diet. This doesn't do them any favors since willpower is like a muscle. At some point, it tires and this is when the dieter goes right back to their old pattern of eating. I have personal experience with this. In terms of health benefits, the keto diet offers the most. The reduction of carbs forces your body to mobilize fat and this results in automatic fat loss and better health.

Feel free to mix and match the recipes you see in here and play around with them. Eating is supposed to be fun! Unfortunately, we've associated fun eating with unhealthy food. This doesn't have to be the case. The air fryer, combined with the Mediterranean diet, will make your mealtimes fun-filled again and full of taste. There's no grease and messy cleanups to deal with anymore. Are you excited yet?

You should be! You're about to embark on a journey full of air fried goodness!

Crispy Croutons

Prep + Cook Time: 20 minutes

4 Servings

INGREDIENTS

2 cups bread cubes

2 tbsp butter, melted

1 tsp dried parsley

Garlic salt and black pepper to taste

DIRECTIONS

Mix the cubed bread with butter, parsley, garlic salt, and black pepper until well coated.

Place in the fryer's basket and AirFry for 6-8 minutes at 380 F, shaking once until golden brown.

Use in soups.

Roasted Asparagus with Serrano Ham

Prep + Cook Time: 15 minutes

4 Servings

INGREDIENTS

12 spears asparagus, trimmed

12 Serrano ham slices

¼ cup Parmesan cheese, grated

Salt and black pepper to taste

DIRECTIONS

Preheat air fryer to 350 F.

Season asparagus with salt and black pepper.

Wrap each ham slice around each asparagus spear from one end to the other end to cover completely.

Arrange them on the greased air fryer basket and AirFry for 10 minutes, shaking once or twice throughout cooking.

When ready, scatter with Parmesan cheese and serve immediately.

Very Berry Breakfast Puffs

Prep + Cook Time: 20 minutes

4 Servings

INGREDIENTS

1 puff pastry sheet

1 tbsp strawberries, mashed

1 tbsp raspberries, mashed

¼ tsp vanilla extract

1 cup cream cheese 1 tbsp honey

DIRECTIONS

Preheat air fryer to 375 F.

Roll the puff pastry out on a lightly floured surface into a 1-inch thick rectangle.

Cut into 4 squares.

Spread the cream cheese evenly on them.

In a bowl, combine the berries, honey, and vanilla.

Spoon the mixture onto the pastry squares.

Fold in the sides over the filling.

Pinch the ends to form a puff.

Place the puffs on a lined with waxed paper baking dish.

Bake in the air fryer for 15 minutes until the pastry is puffed and golden all over.

Let it cool for 10 mins before serving.

Chicken Sun-dried Tomatoes & Mushrooms

Preparation Time: 10 minutes

Cooking Time: 30 minutes

Serve: 4

Ingredients:

2 lbs chicken breasts, halved

8 oz mushrooms, sliced

1/2 cup mayonnaise

1/3 cup sun-dried tomatoes

1 tsp salt

Directions:

Place chicken breasts into the baking dish and top with sun-dried tomatoes, mushrooms, mayonnaise, and salt.

Mix well.

Select Bake mode.

Set time to 30 minutes and temperature 400 F then press START.

The air fryer display will prompt you to ADD FOOD once the temperature is reached then place the baking dish in the air fryer basket.

Serve and enjoy.

BBQ Meatloaf

Preparation Time: 10 minutes

Cooking Time: 35 minutes

Serve: 8

Ingredients:

1 egg 1 tsp chili powder

1 tsp garlic powder

1 tsp garlic, minced

1 tbsp onion, minced

2 lbs ground turkey

2 oz BBQ sauce, sugar-free

1 tsp ground mustard

1 cup cheddar cheese, shredded

1 tsp salt

Directions:

In a large bowl, combine together all ingredients then transfer to the greased casserole dish.

Select Bake mode.

Set time to 35 minutes and temperature 400 F then press START.

The air fryer display will prompt you to ADD FOOD once the temperature is reached then place a casserole dish in the air fryer basket.

Serve and enjoy.

Delicious Chicken Fajita Casserole

Preparation Time: 10 minutes

Cooking Time: 15 minutes

Serve: 4

Ingredients:

1 lb cooked chicken, shredded

1 bell pepper, sliced

1/3 cup mayonnaise

7 oz cream cheese

7 oz cheese, shredded

2 tbsp tex-mix seasoning

1 onion, sliced

Pepper

Salt

Directions:

Mix all ingredients except 2 oz shredded cheese in a greased baking dish.

Spread remaining cheese on top.

Select Bake mode.

Set time to 15 minutes and temperature 400 F then press START.

The air fryer display will prompt you to ADD FOOD once the temperature is reached then place the baking dish in the air fryer basket.

Serve and enjoy.

Creamy Spinach

Preparation Time: 10 minutes

Cooking Time: 20 minutes

Serve: 6

Ingredients:

1lb fresh spinach

1 tbsp onion, minced

8 oz cream cheese

6 oz gouda cheese, shredded

1 tsp garlic powder

Pepper

Salt

Directions:

Spray a large pan with cooking spray and heat over medium heat.

Add spinach to the pan and cook until wilted.

Add cream cheese, garlic powder, and onion and stir until cheese is melted.

Remove pan from heat and add Gouda cheese and season with pepper and salt.

Transfer spinach mixture into the greased baking dish.

Select Bake mode.

Set time to 20 minutes and temperature 400 F then press START.

The air fryer display will prompt you to ADD FOOD once the temperature is reached then place the baking dish in the air fryer basket. Serve and enjoy.

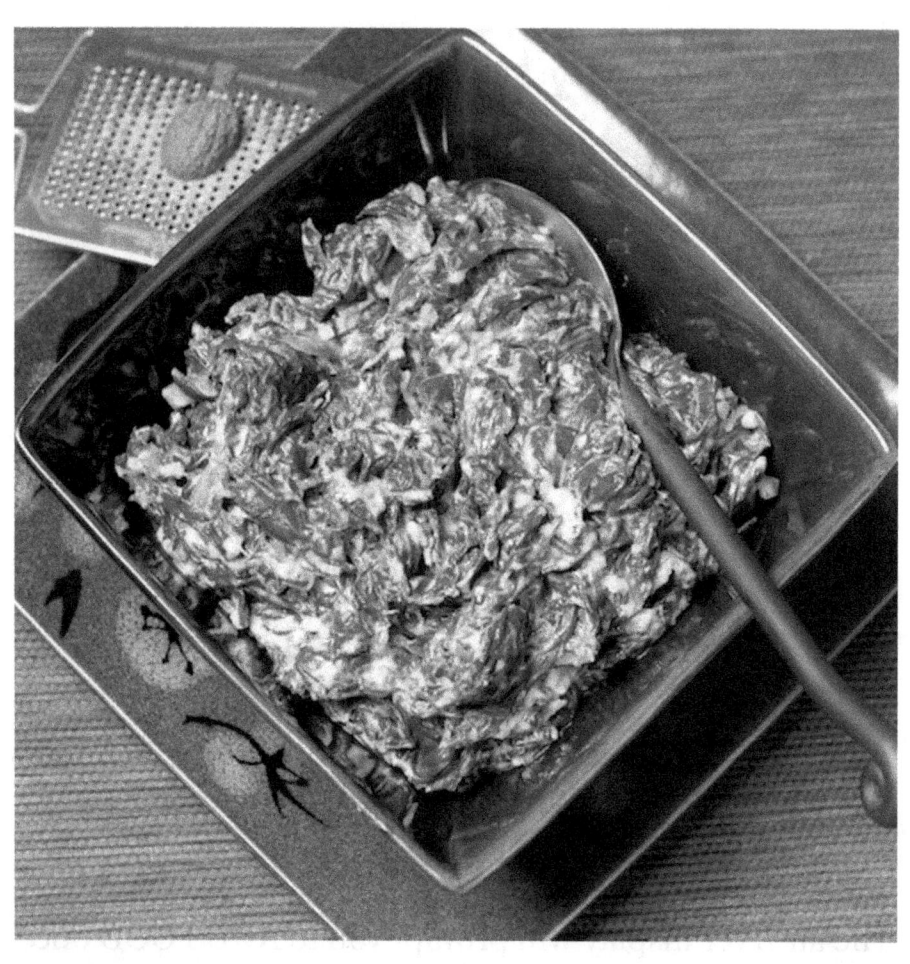

Broccoli Nuggets

Preparation Time: 10 minutes

Cooking Time: 20 minutes

Serve: 4

Ingredients:

2 cups broccoli florets, cooked until soften

1/4 cup almond flour

2 egg whites

1 cup cheddar cheese, shredded

1/8 tsp salt

Directions:

Add cooked broccoli florets into the large bowl and using potato masher mash into small pieces.

Add remaining ingredients into the bowl and mix until well combined.

Make small nuggets from the broccoli mixture.

Select Bake mode.

Set time to 20 minutes and temperature 350 F then press START.

The air fryer display will prompt you to ADD FOOD once the temperature is reached then place broccoli nuggets in the air fryer basket.

Serve and enjoy.

Cauliflower Tomato Rice

Preparation Time: 10 minutes

Cooking Time: 15 minutes

Serve: 3

Ingredients:

1 cauliflower head, cut into florets

1 tomato, chopped

1 onion, chopped

2 tbsp tomato paste

2 tbsp olive oil

1 tsp white pepper

1 tsp black pepper

1 tbsp dried thyme

2 chilies, chopped

2 garlic cloves, chopped

1/2 tsp salt

Directions:

Add cauliflower florets into the food processor and process until it looks like rice.

Stir in tomato paste, tomatoes, and spices and mix well.

Spread cauliflower mixture into the baking dish and drizzle with olive oil.

Select Bake mode.

Set time to 15 minutes and temperature 400 F then press START.

The air fryer display will prompt you to ADD FOOD once the temperature is reached then place the baking dish in the air fryer basket.

Serve and enjoy.

Cheesy Zucchini Noodles

Preparation Time: 10 minutes

Cooking Time: 45 minutes

Serve: 3

Ingredients:

1 egg

2 medium zucchini, trimmed and spiralized

1/2 cup parmesan cheese, grated

1/2 cup feta cheese, crumbled

2 tbsp olive oil

1 cup mozzarella cheese, grated

1 tbsp thyme

1 garlic clove, chopped

1 onion, chopped

1/2 tsp pepper

1/2 tsp salt

Directions:

Add spiralized zucchini and salt in a colander and set aside for 10 minutes.

Gently wash zucchini noodles and pat dry with a paper towel.

Heat oil in a pan over medium heat.

Add garlic and onion and sauté for 3-4 minutes.

Add zucchini noodles and cook for 4 minutes or until softened.

Add zucchini mixture into a baking dish add the eggs, thyme, cheeses.

Mix well and season with pepper and salt.

Select Bake mode.

Set time to 45 minutes and temperature 375 F then press START.

The air fryer display will prompt you to ADD FOOD once the temperature is reached then place the baking dish in the air fryer basket.

Serve and enjoy.

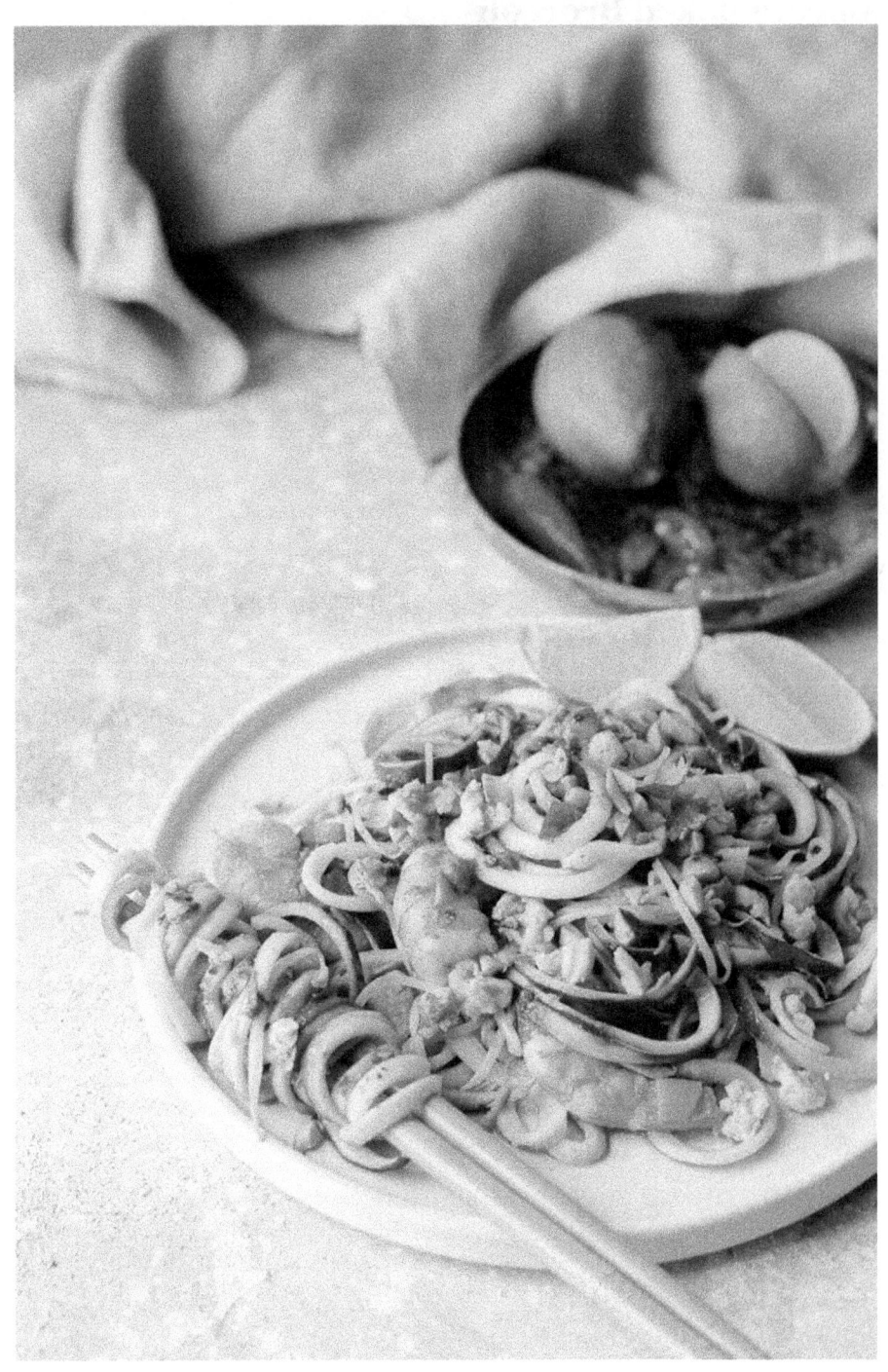

Cheese Baked Broccoli

Preparation Time: 10 minutes

Cooking Time: 10 minutes

Serve: 4

Ingredients:

1 lb broccoli, cut into florets

1/2 cup mozzarella cheese, shredded

1/2 cup heavy cream

2 garlic cloves, minced

1/4 cup parmesan cheese, grated

1/2 cup gruyere cheese, shredded

1 tbsp butter

Directions:

Melt butter in a pan over medium heat.

Add broccoli and season with pepper and salt.

Cook broccoli over medium heat for 5 minutes or until tender.

Add garlic and stir for a minute.

Transfer broccoli into the baking dish.

Pour heavy cream over broccoli then top with parmesan cheese, gruyere cheese, and mozzarella cheese.

Select Bake mode.

Set time to 10 minutes and temperature 375 F then press START.

The air fryer display will prompt you to ADD FOOD once the temperature is reached then place the baking dish in the air fryer basket. Serve and enjoy

Stuffed Bell Peppers

Preparation Time: 10 minutes

Cooking Time: 45 minutes

Serve: 4

Ingredients:

4 eggs

2 medium bell peppers, sliced in half and remove seeds

1/2 cup parmesan cheese, grated

1/2 cup mozzarella cheese, shredded

1/2 cup ricotta cheese

1/4 cup baby spinach

1/4 tsp dried parsley

1 tsp garlic powder

Directions:

Add three cheeses, parsley, garlic powder, and eggs in food processor and process until combined.

Pour egg mixture into each pepper half and top with baby spinach.

Place stuffed peppers in a baking dish.

Cover dish with foil.

Select Bake mode.

Set time to 45 minutes and temperature 375 F then press START.

The air fryer display will prompt you to ADD FOOD once the temperature is reached then place the baking dish in the air fryer basket.

Serve and enjoy.

Delicious Zucchini Casserole

Preparation Time: 10 minutes

Cooking Time: 30 minutes

Serve: 6

Ingredients:

3 medium zucchini, sliced into 1/4-inch thick slices

1 tbsp butter

2 tbsp unsweetened almond milk

1/3 cup heavy cream

3 oz brie cheese

1/2 tbsp Italian seasoning

1 cup Swiss gruyere cheese, shredded

2 garlic cloves, minced

Pepper

Salt

Directions:

Toss zucchini slices with salt and place into a colander and set aside for 45 minutes.

Pat dry with a paper towel.

In a baking dish, arrange zucchini slices and season with pepper and salt.

Combine brie, garlic, butter, almond milk, and cream in a small saucepan and heat for few minutes or until cheese melts.

Pour cheese mixture over zucchini and sprinkle with shredded cheese.

Top with Italian seasoning.

Select Bake mode.

Set time to 30 minutes and temperature 400 F then press START.

The air fryer display will prompt you to ADD FOOD once the temperature is reached then place the baking dish in the air fryer basket.

Serve and enjoy.

Parmesan Squash Casserole

Preparation Time: 10 minutes

Cooking Time: 45 minutes

Serve: 4

Ingredients:

4 medium squash, cut into slices

1/4 cup parmesan cheese, shredded

3/4 stick butter, cut into cubes

1 medium onion, sliced

Pepper

Salt

Directions:

Layer slices squash, onion, butter, pepper, and salt.

Sprinkle with shredded parmesan cheese in a baking dish.

Cover dish with foil.

Select Bake mode.

Set time to 45 minutes and temperature 350 F then press START.

The air fryer display will prompt you to ADD FOOD once the temperature is reached then place the baking dish in the air fryer basket.

Serve and enjoy.

Pecan Green Bean Casserole

Preparation Time: 10 minutes

Cooking Time: 20 minutes

Serve: 4

Ingredients:

1 lb green beans, trimmed and cut into pieces

1/4 cup olive oil

2 oz pecans, crushed

1 small onion, chopped

2 tbsp lemon zest

1/4 cup parmesan cheese, shredded

Directions:

Add all ingredients into the mixing bowl and toss well.

Spread green bean mixture into the baking dish.

Select Bake mode.

Set time to 20 minutes and temperature 400 F then press START.

The air fryer display will prompt you to ADD FOOD once the temperature is reached then place the baking dish in the air fryer basket.

Serve and enjoy

Brussels Sprouts and Broccoli

Preparation Time: 10 minutes

Cooking Time: 30 minutes

Serve: 6

Ingredients:

1 lb broccoli, cut into florets

1 lb Brussels sprouts, cut ends

1 tsp paprika

1/2 onion, chopped

1 tsp garlic powder

1/2 tsp pepper

3 tbsp olive oil

3/4 tsp salt

Directions:

Add all ingredients into the mixing bowl and toss well.

The spread vegetable mixture in a baking dish.

Select Bake mode.

Set time to 30 minutes and temperature 400 F then press START.

The air fryer display will prompt you to ADD FOOD once the temperature is reached then place the baking dish in the air fryer basket.

Serve and enjoy

Basil Eggplant Casserole

Preparation Time: 10 minutes

Cooking Time: 35 minutes

Serve: 6

Ingredients:

1 eggplant, sliced

3 zucchini, sliced

4 tbsp basil, chopped

1 tbsp olive oil

3 garlic cloves, minced

3 oz mozzarella cheese, grated

1/4 cup parsley, chopped

1 cup grape tomatoes, halved

1/4 tsp pepper

1/4 tsp salt

Directions:

Add all ingredients into the large bowl and toss well to combine.

Pour eggplant mixture into the greased baking dish.

Select Bake mode.

Set time to 35 minutes and temperature 350 F then press START.

The air fryer display will prompt you to ADD FOOD once the temperature is reached then place the baking dish in the air fryer basket.

Serve and enjoy.

Spicy Okra

Preparation Time: 10 minutes

Cooking Time: 10 minutes

Serve: 2

Ingredients:

1/2 lb okra, trimmed and sliced

1 tsp olive oil

1/8 tsp pepper

1/2 tsp chili powder

1/2 tsp garlic powder

1/4 tsp salt

Directions:

Add all ingredients into the bowl and toss well.

Select Bake mode.

Set time to 10 minutes and temperature 350 F then press START.

The air fryer display will prompt you to ADD FOOD once the temperature is reached then add okra in the air fryer basket.

Stir halfway through.

Serve and enjoy.

Air Fry Asparagus

Preparation Time: 10 minutes

Cooking Time: 10 minutes

Serve: 4

Ingredients:

1 lb asparagus, ends trimmed and cut in half

1 1/2 tbsp coconut aminos

2 tbsp olive oil

1 tbsp vinegar

Pepper

Salt

Directions:

Add asparagus in a large bowl with remaining ingredients and toss well.

Select Air Fry mode.

Set time to 10 minutes and temperature 400 F then press START.

The air fryer display will prompt you to ADD FOOD once the temperature is reached then place asparagus in the air fryer basket.

Stir halfway through.

Serve and enjoy.

Crisp Brussels Sprouts

Preparation Time: 10 minutes

Cooking Time: 15 minutes

Serve: 4

Ingredients:

2 cups Brussels sprouts

1/4 cup almonds, crushed

1/4 cup parmesan cheese, grated

2 tbsp olive oil

2 tbsp everything bagel seasoning

Salt

Directions:

Add Brussels sprouts into the saucepan with 2 cups of water.

Cover and cook for 8-10 minutes.

Drain well and allow to cool completely.

Sliced each Brussels sprouts in half.

Add Brussels sprouts and remaining ingredients into the mixing bowl and toss to coat.

Select Air Fry mode.

Set time to 15 minutes and temperature 375 F then press START.

The air fryer display will prompt you to ADD FOOD once the temperature is reached then add Brussels sprouts mixture in the air fryer basket.

Serve and enjoy.

Tasty Cauliflower Rice

Preparation Time: 10 minutes

Cooking Time: 40 minutes

Serve: 8

Ingredients:

6 cups grated cauliflower

1/8 tsp red pepper flakes

2 tbsp fresh cilantro, chopped

10 oz can tomatoes with green chilis

1/2 tsp salt

Directions:

Add can tomatoes into the blender and blend well.

Add grated cauliflower, cilantro, tomatoes, red pepper flakes, and salt into the prepared baking dish and stir until well combined.

Select Bake mode.

Set time to 40 minutes and temperature 350 F then press START.

The air fryer display will prompt you to ADD FOOD once the temperature is reached then place the baking dish in the air fryer basket.

Serve and enjoy.

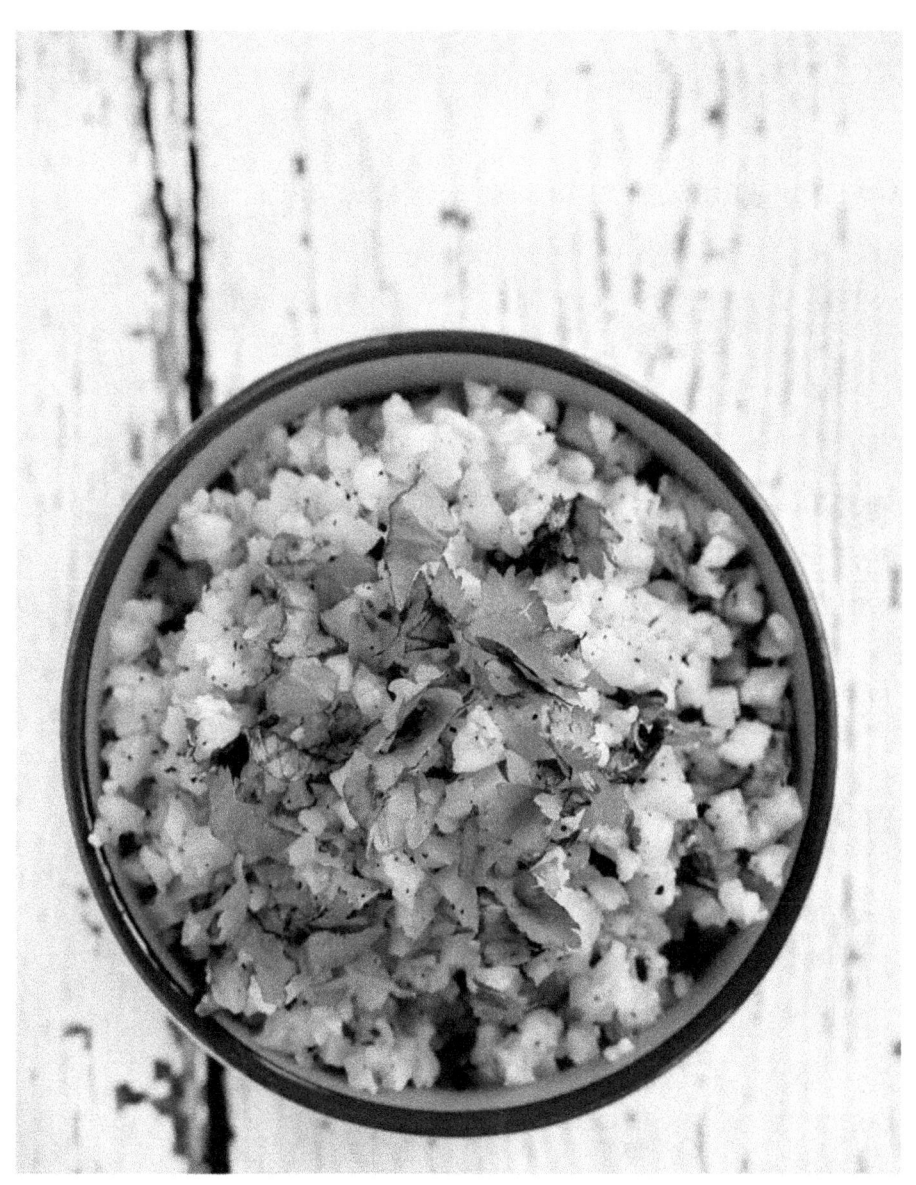

Spinach Squares

Preparation Time: 10 minutes

Cooking Time: 35 minutes

Serve: 9

Ingredients:

3 eggs

1/2 cup ricotta cheese

16 oz frozen spinach, cooked and drained

8 oz cheddar cheese, grated

1/2 tsp paprika

Pepper

Salt

Directions:

Add eggs, paprika, ricotta cheese, pepper, and salt into the blender and blend until smooth.

Stir in spinach and cheese.

Pour egg mixture into the greased baking dish.

Select Bake mode.

Set time to 35 minutes and temperature 350 F then press START.

The air fryer display will prompt you to ADD FOOD once the temperature is reached then place the baking dish in the air fryer basket.

Slice and serve.

Vegetable Kebabs

Preparation Time: 10 minutes

Cooking Time: 10 minutes

Serve: 4

Ingredients:

2 bell peppers, cut into 1-inch pieces

1 eggplant, cut into 1-inch pieces

1/2 onion, cut into 1-inch pieces

1 zucchini, cut into 1-inch pieces

Pepper

Salt

Directions:

Thread vegetables onto the soaked wooden skewers and spray them with cooking spray.

Season with pepper and salt.

Select Air Fry mode.

Set time to 10 minutes and temperature 390 F then press START.

The air fryer display will prompt you to ADD FOOD once the temperature is reached then place skewers in the air fryer basket.

Turn halfway through.

Serve and enjoy.

Blackened Tilapia

Preparation Time: 10 minutes

Cooking Time: 14 minutes

Serve: 3

Ingredients:

3 tilapia fillets

1 tbsp dried parsley flakes

1/4 tsp cayenne pepper

1 tsp garlic powder

1 tsp onion powder

2 1/2 tbsp paprika

1/2 tsp pepper

1 tsp salt

Directions:

In a small bowl, mix together paprika, pepper, onion powder, garlic powder, cayenne, parsley, pepper, and salt.

Spray fish fillets with cooking spray.

Rub the paprika mixture on both sides of fish fillets.

Place the cooking tray in the air fryer basket.

Line air fryer basket with parchment paper.

Select Bake mode.

Set time to 14 minutes and temperature 400 F then press START.

The air fryer display will prompt you to ADD FOOD once the temperature is reached then place the fish fillet in the air fryer basket.

Serve and enjoy.

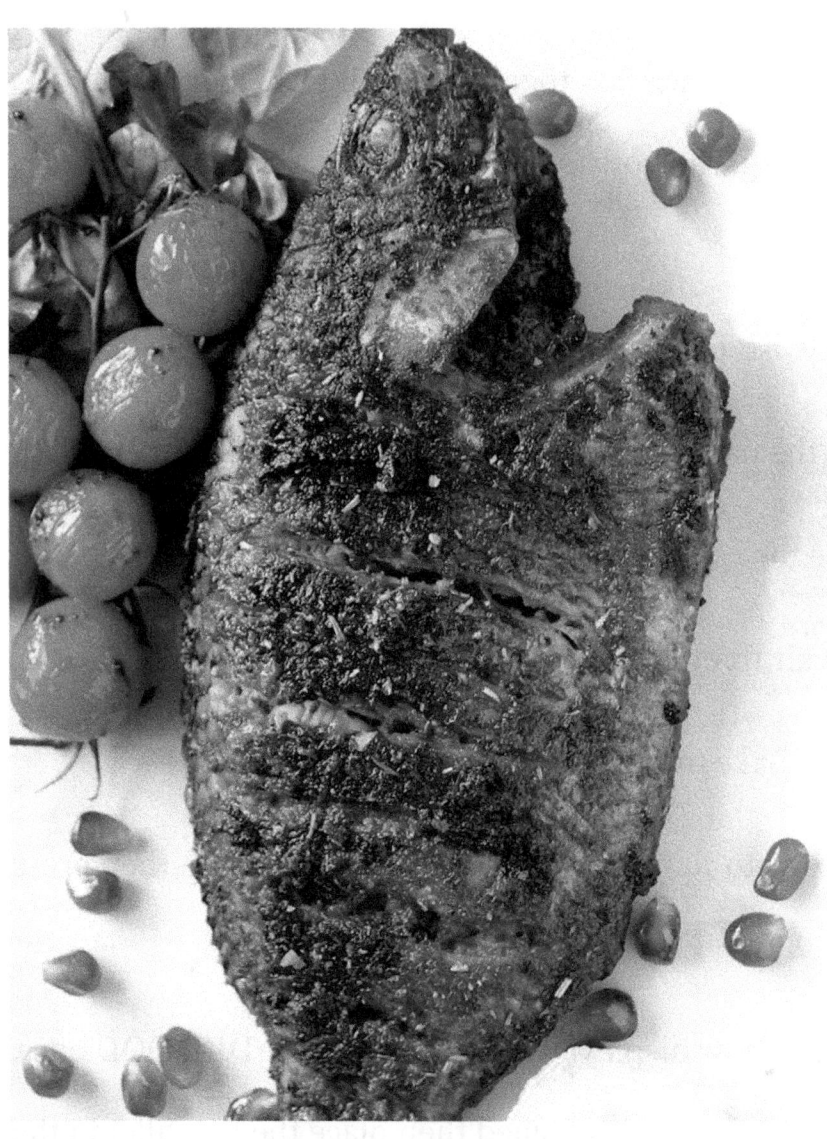

Garlic Butter Baked Shrimp

Preparation Time: 10 minutes

Cooking Time: 8 minutes

Serve: 4

Ingredients:

1 1/2 lbs shrimp, peeled & deveined

1/4 cup parmesan cheese, grated

1/2 tsp paprika

1 tsp garlic powder

1/4 tsp pepper

1/4 cup butter, melted

1 tsp kosher salt

Directions:

Add shrimp and remaining ingredients into the large bowl and toss well.

Place the cooking tray in the air fryer basket.

Line air fryer basket with parchment paper.

Select Bake mode.

Set time to 8 minutes and temperature 400 F then press START.

The air fryer display will prompt you to ADD FOOD once the temperature is reached then add shrimp in the air fryer basket.

Serve and enjoy.

Cajun Catfish Fillets

Preparation Time: 10 minutes

Cooking Time: 25 minutes

Serve: 2

Ingredients:

2 catfish fillets

1/2 tbsp olive oil

1/2 tsp red pepper flakes, crushed

1/2 tsp oregano

1/2 tsp paprika

1/2 tsp cayenne pepper

1/2 tsp onion powder

1/2 tsp garlic powder

Pepper

Salt

Directions:

In a small bowl, mix together garlic powder, onion powder, cayenne pepper, paprika, oregano, red pepper flakes, pepper, and salt.

Brush fish fillets with olive oil and rub with spice mixture.

Place the cooking tray in the air fryer basket.

Line air fryer basket with parchment paper.

Select Bake mode.

Set time to 25 minutes and temperature 350 F then press START.

The air fryer display will prompt you to ADD FOOD once the temperature is reached then place fish fillets in the air fryer basket.

Serve and enjoy.

Lemon Garlic Shrimp

Preparation Time: 10 minutes

Cooking Time: 14 minutes

Serve: 3

Ingredients:

1 lb shrimp, peeled & deveined

1/4 tsp garlic powder

1 tbsp olive oil

1/2 lemon

Pepper

Salt

Directions:

In a mixing bowl, toss shrimp with garlic powder, olive oil, pepper, and salt.

Place the cooking tray in the air fryer basket.

Select Air Fry mode.

Set time to 14 minutes and temperature 400 F then press START.

The air fryer display will prompt you to ADD FOOD once the temperature is reached then add shrimp in the air fryer basket.

Shake basket halfway through.

Squeeze lemon juice over shrimp and serve.

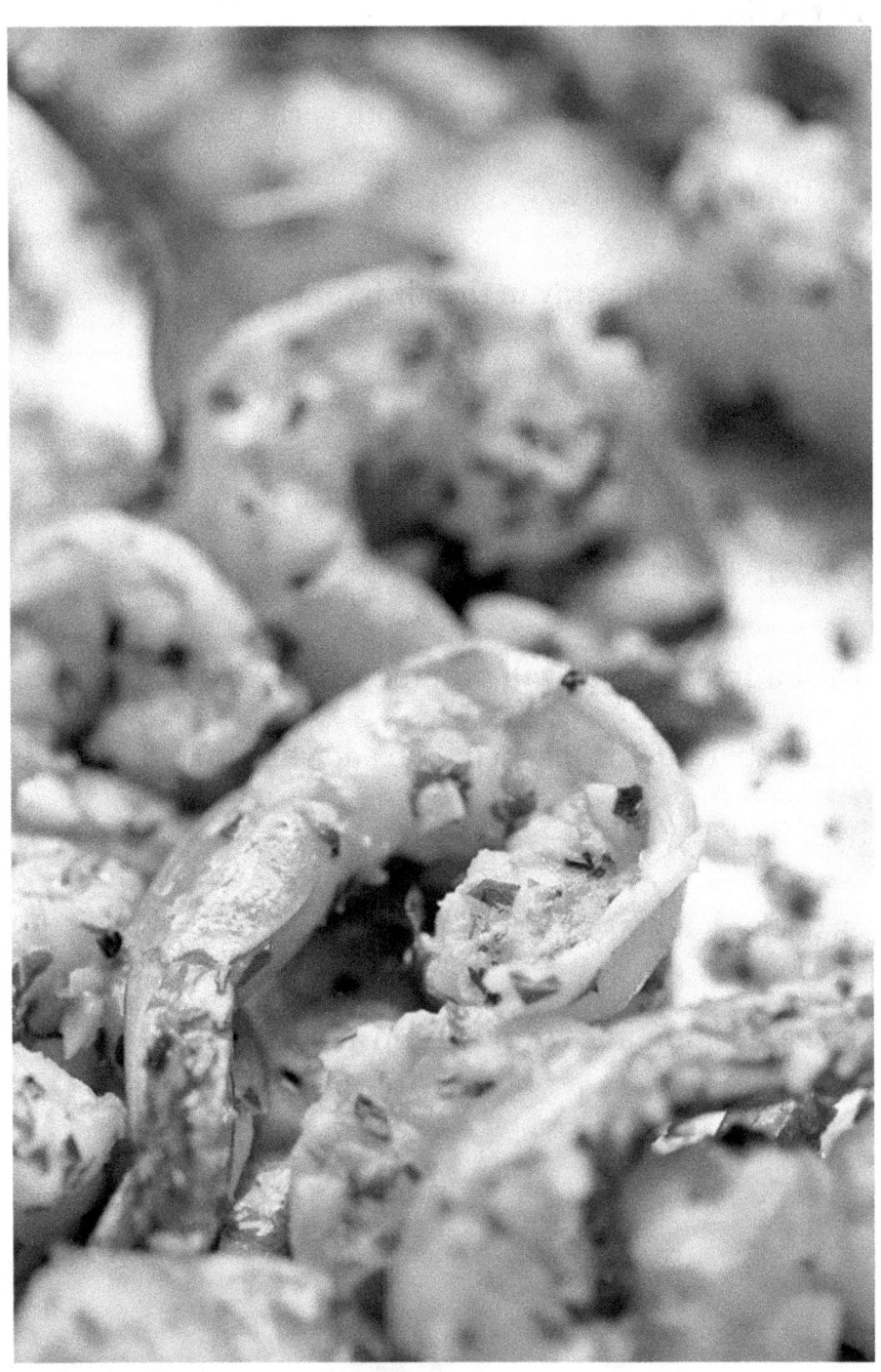

Cod with Vegetables

Preparation Time: 10 minutes

Cooking Time: 15 minutes

Serve: 4

Ingredients:

1 lb cod fillets

1/2 tsp paprika

1/4 cup olive oil

1/4 cup lemon juice

8 oz asparagus, chopped

3 cups broccoli, chopped

1/2 tsp lemon pepper seasoning

1 tsp salt

Directions:

In a small bowl, mix together lemon juice, paprika, olive oil, lemon pepper seasoning, and salt.

Place the cooking tray in the air fryer basket.

Line air fryer basket with parchment paper.

Select Bake mode.

Set time to 15 minutes and temperature 400 F then press START.

The air fryer display will prompt you to ADD FOOD once the temperature is reached.

Then place fish fillets in the middle of the parchment paper in the air fryer basket.

Place broccoli and asparagus around the fish fillets.

Pour lemon juice mixture over the fish fillets.

Serve and enjoy.

Healthy Swordfish Fillets

Preparation Time: 10 minutes

Cooking Time: 20 minutes

Serve: 2

Ingredients:

12 oz swordfish fillets

1 garlic clove, minced

2 tsp fresh parsley, chopped

3 tbsp olive oil

1/2 tsp lemon zest, grated

1/2 tsp ginger, grated

1/8 tsp crushed red pepper

Directions:

In a small bowl, mix together 2 tablespoon oil, lemon zest, red pepper, ginger, garlic, and parsley.

Season fish fillets with salt.

Heat remaining oil in a pan over medium-high heat.

Place fish fillets in the pan and cook until lightly browned 2-3 minutes.

Select Bake mode.

Set time to 10 minutes and temperature 400 F then press START.

The air fryer display will prompt you to ADD FOOD once the temperature is reached then place fish fillets in the air fryer basket.

Pour oil mixture over fish fillets and serve.

Air Fry Fish Patties

Preparation Time: 10 minutes

Cooking Time: 6 minutes

Serve: 4

Ingredients:

1 egg, lightly beaten

1/4 cup almond flour

8 oz can tuna, drained

1 tbsp mustard

Pepper

Salt

Directions:

Add all ingredients into the large bowl and mix until well combined.

Make four equal shapes of patties from the mixture.

Select Air Fry mode.

Set time to 6 minutes and temperature 400 F then press START.

The air fryer display will prompt you to ADD FOOD once the temperature is reached then place patties in the air fryer basket.

Turn patties halfway through.

Serve and enjoy.

Delicious Shrimp Fajitas

Preparation Time: 10 minutes

Cooking Time: 22 minutes

Serve: 12

Ingredients:

1 lb shrimp

1/2 cup onion, diced

2 bell pepper, diced

1 tbsp olive oil

2 tbsp taco seasoning

Directions:

Add shrimp and remaining ingredients into the bowl and toss well.

Select Air Fry mode.

Set time to 22 minutes and temperature 390 F then press START.

The air fryer display will prompt you to ADD FOOD once the temperature is reached then place shrimp mixture in the air fryer basket.

Stir halfway through. Serve and enjoy.

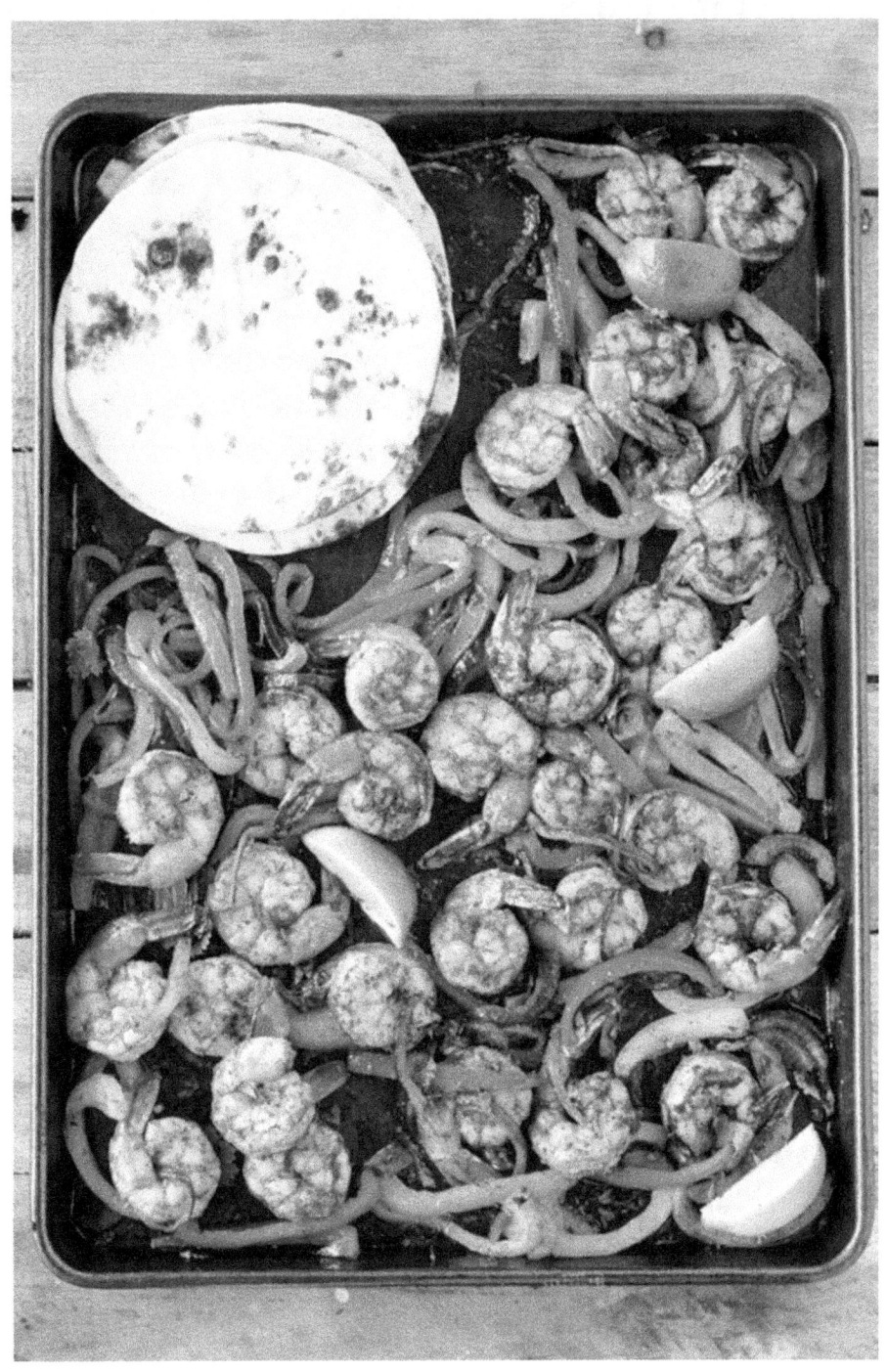

Tasty Crab Patties

Preparation Time: 10 minutes

Cooking Time: 10 minutes

Serve: 4

Ingredients:

8 oz crab meat

2 tbsp mayonnaise

2 green onion, chopped

1/4 cup bell pepper, chopped

1 tsp old bay seasoning

1 tbsp Dijon mustard

2 tbsp almond flour

Pepper

Salt

Directions:

Add all ingredients into the mixing bowl and mix until well combined.

Make 4 equal shapes of patties from the mixture.

Select Air Fry mode.

Set time to 10 minutes and temperature 370 F then press START.

The air fryer display will prompt you to ADD FOOD once the temperature is reached then place patties in the air fryer basket.

Serve and enjoy.

Cajun Scallops

Preparation Time: 10 minutes

Cooking Time: 6 minutes

Serve: 1

Ingredients:

4 scallops, rinsed and pat dry

1/2 tsp Cajun seasoning

Pepper

Salt

Directions:

Spray scallops with cooking spray and season with Cajun seasoning, pepper, and salt.

Select Air Fry mode.

Set time to 6 minutes and temperature 400 F then press START.

The air fryer display will prompt you to ADD FOOD once the temperature is reached then place scallops in the air fryer basket.

Turn scallops halfway through.

Serve and enjoy.

Greek Baked Salmon

Preparation Time: 10 minutes

Cooking Time: 20 minutes

Serve: 5

Ingredients:

1 3/4 lbs salmon fillet

1/3 cup artichoke hearts

1/4 cup sun-dried tomatoes, drained

1/4 cup olives, pitted and chopped

1/3 cup basil pesto

1 tbsp fresh dill, chopped

1/4 cup capers

1 tsp paprika

1/4 tsp salt

Directions:

Season salmon with paprika and salt.

Place the cooking tray in the air fryer basket.

Place piece of parchment paper into the air fryer basket.

Select Bake mode.

Set time to 20 minutes and temperature 400 F then press START.

The air fryer display will prompt you to ADD FOOD once the temperature is reached then place salmon in the air fryer basket and top with remaining ingredients.

Serve and enjoy.

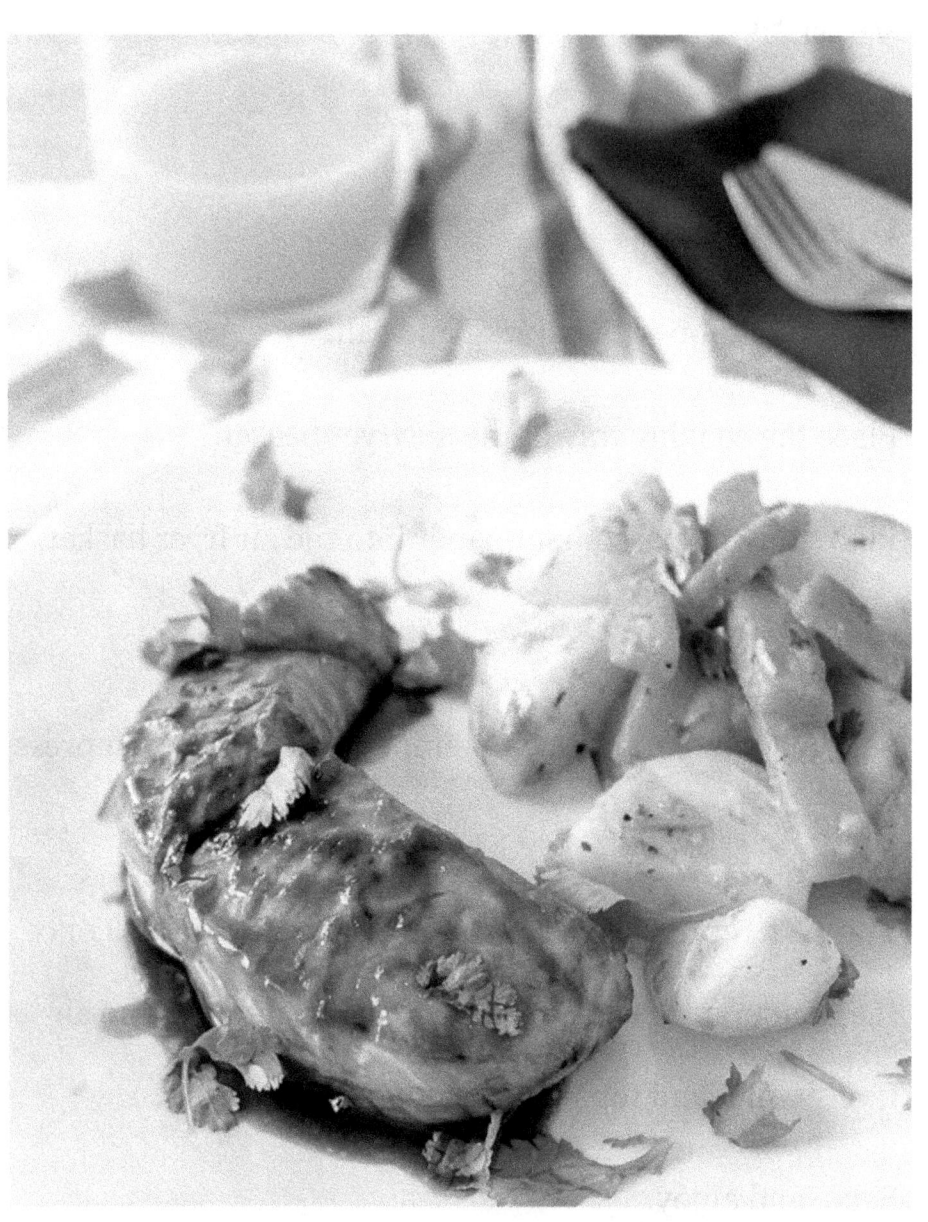

White Fish Fillet with Roasted Pepper

Preparation Time: 10 minutes

Cooking Time: 30 minutes

Serve: 1

Ingredients:

8 oz frozen white fish fillet

1/2 tsp Italian seasoning

1 1/2 tbsp butter, melted

1 tbsp lemon juice

1 tbsp fresh parsley, chopped

1 tbsp roasted red bell pepper, diced

Directions:

Place the fish fillet in a baking dish.

Drizzle butter and lemon juice over fish.

Sprinkle with Italian seasoning.

Top with roasted bell pepper and parsley.

Select Bake mode.

Set time to 30 minutes and temperature 400 F then press START.

The air fryer display will prompt you to ADD FOOD once the temperature is reached then place the baking dish in the air fryer basket.

Serve and enjoy

Rosemary Basil Salmon

Preparation Time: 10 minutes

Cooking Time: 15 minutes

Serve: 4

Ingredients:

1 lbs salmon, cut into 4 pieces

1 tbsp olive oil

1/2 tbsp dried rosemary

1/4 tsp dried basil

1 tbsp dried chives

Pepper Salt

Directions:

Mix together olive oil, basil, chives, and rosemary.

Brush salmon with oil mixture.

Select Air Fry mode.

Set time to 15 minutes and temperature 400 F then press START.

The air fryer display will prompt you to ADD FOOD once the temperature is reached then place salmon pieces in the air fryer basket.

Serve and enjoy.

Tomato Basil Fish Fillets

Preparation Time: 10 minutes

Cooking Time: 20 minutes

Serve: 2

Ingredients:

2 salmon fillets

1 tomato, sliced

1 tbsp dried basil

2 tbsp parmesan cheese, grated

1 tbsp olive oil

Directions:

Place salmon fillets in the baking dish.

Sprinkle basil on top of salmon fillets.

Arrange tomato slices on top of salmon fillets.

Drizzle with oil and sprinkle cheese on top.

Select Bake mode.

Set time to 20 minutes and temperature 375 F then press START.

The air fryer display will prompt you to ADD FOOD once the temperature is reached then place the baking dish in the air fryer basket.

Serve and enjoy.

Baked Salmon & Carrots

Preparation Time: 10 minutes

Cooking Time: 20 minutes

Serve: 4

Ingredients:

1 lb salmon, cut into four pieces

2 tbsp olive oil

2 cups baby carrots

Salt

Directions:

Place salmon pieces in the baking dish.

In a mixing bowl, toss together baby carrots and olive oil.

Arrange carrot around the salmon.

Select Bake mode.

Set time to 20 minutes and temperature 400 F then press START.

The air fryer display will prompt you to ADD FOOD once the temperature is reached then place the baking dish in the air fryer basket.

Serve and enjoy.

Baked Shrimp Scampi

Preparation Time: 10 minutes

Cooking Time: 13 minutes

Serve: 4

Ingredients:

1 lb shrimp, peeled and deveined

1/4 cup parmesan cheese, grated

8 garlic cloves, peeled

2 tbsp olive oil

1 fresh lemon, cut into wedges

Directions:

Add all ingredients except parmesan cheese into the mixing bowl and toss well.

Transfer shrimp mixture into the baking dish.

Select Bake mode.

Set time to 13 minutes and temperature 400 F then press START.

The air fryer display will prompt you to ADD FOOD once the temperature is reached then place the baking dish in the air fryer basket.

Sprinkle with parmesan cheese and serve.

Tangy Salmon

Preparation Time: 10 minutes

Cooking Time: 22 minutes

Serve: 4

Ingredients:

2 lbs salmon fillet, skinless and boneless

1 tbsp olive oil

1/4 cup fresh dill

1 chili, sliced

2 fresh lemon juice

1 orange juice

Pepper

Salt

Directions:

Place salmon fillet in a baking dish and drizzle with olive oil, lemon juice, and orange juice.

Sprinkle chili over the salmon and season with pepper and salt.

Select Bake mode. Set time to 22 minutes and temperature 350 F then press START.

The air fryer display will prompt you to ADD FOOD once the temperature is reached then place the baking dish in the air fryer basket.

Garnish with dill.

Serve and enjoy.

Cheese Herb Salmon

Preparation Time: 10 minutes

Cooking Time: 10 minutes

Serve: 5

Ingredients:

5 salmon fillets

1/4 cup fresh parsley, chopped

3 garlic cloves, minced

3/4 cup parmesan cheese, shredded

1 tsp McCormick's BBQ seasoning

1 tsp paprika

1 tbsp olive oil

Pepper

Salt

Directions:

Add salmon, seasoning, and olive oil to the bowl and mix well.

Place salmon fillet into the baking dish.

In a bowl, mix together cheese, garlic, and parsley.

Sprinkle cheese mixture on top of salmon.

Select Air Fry mode.

Set time to 10 minutes and temperature 400 F then press START.

The air fryer display will prompt you to ADD FOOD once the temperature is reached then place the baking dish in the air fryer basket.

Serve and enjoy.

Crispy Coconut Shrimp

Preparation Time: 10 minutes

Cooking Time: 5 minutes

Serve: 4

Ingredients:

2 egg whites

16 oz shrimp, peeled

1/2 cup shredded coconut

1/2 cup almond flour

1/2 tsp salt

Directions:

Whisk egg whites in a shallow dish.

In a bowl, mix together shredded coconut and almond flour.

Dip shrimp into the egg then coat with coconut mixture.

Select Air Fry mode.

Set time to 5 minutes and temperature 400 F then press START.

The air fryer display will prompt you to ADD FOOD once the temperature is reached then place coated shrimp in the air fryer basket.

Serve and enjoy

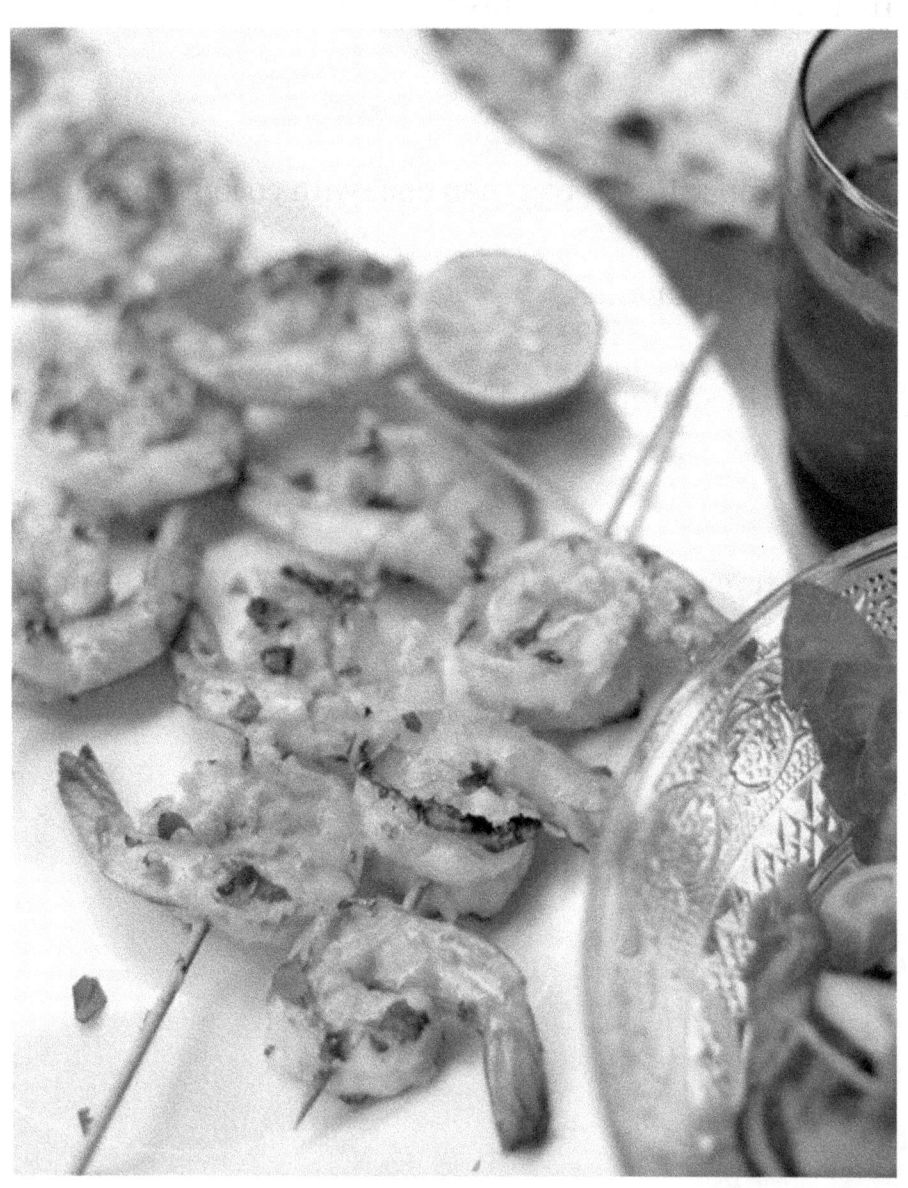

www.ingramcontent.com/pod-product-compliance
Lightning Source LLC
Chambersburg PA
CBHW071110030426
42336CB00013BA/2021